Intermittent Fasting for Men

In 5 Minutes

KRIS TRELSKI

ISBN: 9781699905692

To my wife Halina and my sons Mike, Tom, Greg and Jacek who inspired me to write this book, don't even know that I did, and probably will never read it. I love you guys.

CONTENTS

Intermittent Fasting for Men

ACKNOWLEDGMENTS

I would like to thank my wife who noticed quite early that I am losing weight and for patiently understanding my insistence on continuing to do something we are not supposed to.

INTRODUCTION

About 5 months ago I hated getting on the scale because I knew that nothing was changing, I was stuck at the high number of about 240 pounds and nothing I did would change that. But I did stick to my plan and kept crawling onto the scale anyway. Finally, I started to see small changes. From week to week the scale started to go down by a pound on average. It wasn't that much. Usually that's something that would self-correct by gaining 2 pounds, but not this time. Then the difference increased to 2 pounds per week. That was fine with me if it continued, and it did. From that point my weight numbers were going only one way, down.

HOW IT ALL STARTED

Several years ago, I started a diet and exercise program based on books I have read. I lost about 10 pounds and was very happy and proud of myself. For exercise I used Negatives (*) and for dieting, I used two methods. In one I counted the calories in each of my meals. At some point I also added the time frame (second method) when I would eat. I did that after reading an article about Terry Crews, the "most ripped man" in Hollywood. I decided to only eat between 10 am and 10 pm. I was sure, however, that my success was due to counting those calories.

Then it happened. After some difficult events in my life I stopped following my weight loss program and started to re-gain weight. Slowly but firmly. To the point where I weighted more than ever before.

* Links to the book(s) and/or accessories are available on my website, fasting4men.com.

FOUNDATION FOR A CHANGE

Over a year ago, my life was as plain as it could get. I worked 40-hour week and then I drove for Uber over the weekends. I was going to the gym 3 times a week, but I did not see any improvement either in my weight or posture. I was officially, my doctor told me, obese.

Then, a wonderful thing happened. We bought two dogs, warm and fuzzy Sheepadoodles. — FOUNDATION BLOCK #1

That meant that someone had to walk those dogs, and they were bigger and stronger than most dogs, at least twice a day for about 30 minutes each. Obviously, that was a task I loved to do.

Then, as a present, I got a Fitbit watch so I could keep track of my walks. That was fun, but then I found even better Fitbit accessory, an electronic weight scale that keeps track of my weight and body fat.

I could now watch my progress on my phone and/or on a personal Fitbit webpage. — FOUNDATION BLOCK #2

ENTER TERRY

On May 21, 2019, I came across "100 Pushups A Day For 30 Days Challenge" on YouTube. I took it to my heart. I knew that I can do it and kept doing it. Sometimes if I forgot to do it during the day, I would do 60, 80 or even 100 pushups right before going to bed. As you would have guessed nothing happened. Nothing! Being 58 just sucks. But I did feel stronger. So, I started my own "200 Pushups A Day For 30 Days Challenge." This time I also added an Intermittent Fasting.

Why did I add the Fasting? Again, it was because of Terry Crew's videos on YouTube. Among them, "Terry Crews - 4% Body Fat at 50! | Body Transformation." That's exact title, find it, watch it because almost at the end he mentions how he eats. Have I not watched the whole video, and trust me, I got a little bit tired around 8th minute, I would have not lost those 35 pounds.

I found Terry entertaining and, should I say, down to earth, so I believed what he said. While I don't think I will ever do 2-hour workout in the gym, I do work for a living, I did increase my time there from 40 minutes to one hour. And, I work out every day, Monday to Friday with Wednesday being a special workout day.

I trusted Terry enough that I started his version of intermittent fasting 16:8. Except, unlike his schedule of 2pm-10pm, it was easier for me to do it from noon to 8pm. I don't think I would ever make it to 2pm. Many times, I don't even make it to noon. I usually start at 11:50 am.

WHAT IS INTERMITTENT FASTING?

Intermittent Fasting is considered by many people a dietary revolution not only because of the benefits it allegedly brings, but also because it undermines many of the principles of healthy eating that have been taught to us so far.

According to Wikipedia Intermittent Fasting (intermittent energy restriction or intermittent calorie restriction) is an umbrella term for various eating diet plans that cycle between a period of fasting and non-fasting over a defined period.

Three methods of intermittent fasting are: alternate-day fasting, whole-day fasting, and time-restricted feeding.

- Alternate day fasting (ADF) is the strictest form of intermittent fasting. This involves 24-hours complete fasting followed by a 24-hour non-fasting period. There is an adjusted form of ADF which allows the consumption of approximately 25% of daily calorie needs on fasting days instead of full fasting.

- Whole day fasting involves regular one or two fasting days per week. As an example, 5:2 diets require five non-fasting days and 2 fasting days in a week. During the fasting days, it allows approximately 500 to 600 calories or about 25% of regular daily caloric intake.

- Time-restricted feeding involves eating only during a certain number of hours each day. A good example can be 16:8 diet which advocate 16 fasting hours cycled by 8 non-fasting hours. There are also, 12:12 and 20:4 (20 fasting and 4 feeding).

To sum it all up, all ways to do intermittent fasting split the day or week into eating and fasting periods. But many people find the Time-restricted Feeding, especially the 16:8 method, to be the simplest, most sustainable and easiest to stick to. It's also the most popular.

The first introduction of Time-restricted Feeding to the general public was in 2002 in Hofmekler's Warrior Diet. It proposes 4-6 hours of feeding and 20-18 hours of either under-feeding or simply fasting. The author of the Warrior Diet argues that since our ancestors hunted, fought or worked nearly 20 hours a day and then fed at night it should be easy for us to follow it since we already have it imprinted in our genes.

Intermittent fasting using the 16:8 method means limiting the consumption of foods and drinks containing calories to a fixed window for eight hours a day and abstaining from food for the remaining 16 hours. It is generally thought to be less restrictive and more flexible than many other diet plans and can easily adapt to any lifestyle.

16:8 method – rules:
Start by choosing an eight-hour window and limit your food intake until then. Many people prefer to eat from

noon to 20:00, because this means that you only need to fast at night and skip breakfast, but you can still eat a balanced lunch and dinner, as well as a few snacks throughout the day. Others decide to eat from 9am to 5pm, which allows for a healthy breakfast around 9am, a normal lunch around noon and a light early dinner or snack around 4pm before the start of the fast.

Regardless of when you eat, it is recommended to eat several small meals and snacks evenly spaced throughout the day to help stabilize blood sugar levels and keep hunger under control. In addition, to maximize the potential health benefits of your diet, it's important to eat whole foods and drinks while eating.

This is very important because eating unhealthy foods, making up or eating in reserve can cause weight gain and promote the development of many diseases, including eating disorders.

Although 16:8 intermittent fasting is generally considered safe for most healthy adults, it's worth talking to your doctor before starting (even if it is to make him aware of what you are up to). It' important especially if we are struggling with chronic diseases and taking various medications.

What do researchers think about 16:8 method?
In a study that appeared in the journal on nutrition and healthy aging, researchers confirmed that this type of fasting can effectively help people with obesity lose weight. Study participants who followed this plan for 12 weeks lost 3 percent of their total body weight at the end of the study period. Also, the 16:8 diet style helped them maintain lower

blood pressure. This is important because obesity is a major risk factor for hypertension, which can lead to more serious cardiovascular problems.

Another study, published in the journal on obesity, suggested that intermittent fasting could have many other health benefits. Its authors say that this diet style works by changing metabolism. Fasting periods propel the body to start burning fat, not sugars, to convert it into the energy we need. This makes intermittent fasting so effective in losing weight. However, the authors also speculate that metabolic processes triggered by this type of diet can also increase life expectancy, protect cognitive function, and reduce inflammation.

Many studies have found the relationship between obesity and the increased risk of developing certain types of cancer. Now, the latest reports also say that Intermittent Fasting can be an effective cancer prevention strategy. They suggest that instead of, or besides, changing your diet, it may be important to simply pay attention to time you eat your meals.

Studies in mice have shown that time-limited eating can stop tumor growth. In addition, researchers found some mechanisms that could explain the relationship between obesity and cancer.

Research results revealed, among others, that obese mice on time-limited diets experienced significantly less tumor growth than mice that ate without restrictions.

As it was mentioned above this diet also helps fight inflammation. Inflammation is a defense mechanism that helps fight various infections in the body. Unfortunately, our eating habits promote excessive inflammation. Experts say that many people struggle with numerous inflammations because they eat too much and too often.

Inflammation can lead to various diseases such as diabetes, multiple sclerosis and inflammatory bowel syndrome. Intermittent Fasting can help in the fight against them.

The reduction in a risk of inflammation was found to be due to a reduction in the number of cells in the blood, called 'monocytes', that cause inflammation.

Several well know people are known to be on Intermittent Fasting, among them: Terry Crews, Hugh Jackman, Justin Theroux 12-12, and Benedict Cumberbatch 5-2.

MY FASTING PLAN

Before I will make a recommendation for your diet plan. I would like to tell you about mine.

When I started my Intermittent Fasting, I did not change anything in my diet except for the eating and no-eating periods, basically I reversed them. You read it right, previously my eating period was matching the hours (16-18) I did not sleep. That does not mean that I ate constantly. I just did not have any problem having a snack right before I went to bed.

It started with an experimental period, but I quickly settled on 12 noon – 8 pm period. It was mostly for a convenience of not having to spend time on figuring out what should I eat for breakfast or 10 am snack time. I must confess that in the beginning, it was a little difficult and many times I started eating at around 11:45. The best way to fight that was to find something really, really important to do to get my mind off of it. On the other hand, having my last meal before 8 pm was not a problem. Sometimes, I simply stuffed myself on purpose around 7 pm.

The funny thing is, I quickly stopped eating Mc Donald's food. I simply didn't feel a need for it. Also, I started to pay closer attention to calorie counts on the menu and found that eating 900-1100 calories in one meal is way too much. On the other hand, I have now begun to allow myself to have a slice of pepperoni pizza once a week.

Having an electronic scale that records my daily weight measurements helps me monitor which foods cause me to gain a pound or two from day to day. That way, I have to say, I was successful in dropping at least a pound every week.

As I just said, Fitbit scale lets me identify foods that may cause trouble for me and sabotage my diet. For example, I love Polish food so I would often buy a takeout from Polish restaurant. Unfortunately, Polish food is high in calories and to make things worse the restaurant sells the meals so big that they could feed another person. Ok, maybe half a person or a skinny one, but still I must keep it in mind. Now I simply leave some of it on a plate.

So, what do I eat now and how much? When, the clock hits 12:00 noon I start with a few pretzels. Then I have some fruit and yogurt. Sometime later I have a small sandwich or simply a slice of cranberry-and-nuts bread with butter. Sometime later I will have a fistful of nuts. For my largest meal I will have either a turkey sandwich, or a soup.

Many diet books have pages upon pages of meals that make my pop and hair stand-up. Mostly because I never heard of many of them and they look very strange and unappetizing.

I cannot give you any recipes of my own because when I cook, I go by what is in the fridge and what I will come up with.

FASTING PLAN FOR YOU

First, I recommend the Time-restricted Feeding, 16:8, other combinations are fine too. For example, 12:12 is great if you want to maintain your weight and a healthy lifestyle. Once you select one, stick to it for the first week. It's the same as with committing to the gym membership, all you must do for a first couple of weeks is to show up.

Make sure that the times you picked work for you. While you are at it, you should also set your sleep schedule so your internal (body) clock is set and works for you and not against.

In the first few weeks you do not have to make any diet changes, unless you feel like it.

When, you feel comfortable with the schedule, let's say 11am to 7pm, you can start modifying your diet. But that is entirely up to you.

Let's take a closer look at your fasting/eating periods and let's use 16/8 as an example. The fasting period will last 16 hours and eating period will be 8 hours, but since we need to sleep, let's make sure that our sleep is in the 16 hour period, which basically means that if you sleep for 8 hours your actual fasting period is only 8 hours. Don't forget that during the fasting period you can drink (non-caloric) fluids and that includes coffee (low-fat milk and no-sugar). Finally, in your 16-hour fasting period you can do any form of exercise or just go to the gym and workout as much as you can handle. Some people say that because of fasting you may feel weaker and your workout will not be as good as it should. I can say with certainty that I never felt better than working out hungry. I never felt any hunger while exercising. Obviously, drinking Gatorade while in the gym may have helped since it's a 200-calorie drink (after a while I started to water it down).

As I said, you can practically eat anything you want, but please watch the sugar. This is the only factor that can sabotage your efforts. Try to limit it as much as possible.

So, basically this is it. Don't be afraid to experiment with your diet. After 3 or more months of Intermittent Fasting you will have all the rights to do so.

When you successfully lose weight people will notice and you may be asked to help others by going on diet with them. It is perfectly fine to do so, but do not allow yourself to be bullied into quitting your IF just because the other diet doesn't require eating/fasting periods.

For example, I am being pressed to provide someone with support doing a very demanding Dabrowska Diet, which is actually a Polish version of fasting where fasting occurs because you only eat fresh fruit and vegetables (some, not all) and you simply can't eat more than 800 calories of food a day, it's simply impossible to pass that number. My condition was that I am staying on my eating plan and it was accepted.

Again, this diet is about your eating and fasting times. It is just that simple and hard as well. If you stick to it for more than 2 months you will succeed.

ABOUT THE AUTHOR

Kris lives with his family in Connecticut. His other passions are history of Warsaw Uprising and Yoga. He is an author of "Killing Warsaw: The Facts About Warsaw Uprising" and "Yoga for Men in 5 Minutes." You can find him at Fasting4men.com or FortisYoga.com.

9 781699 905692